MW01233984

The Complete Mediterranean Diet Cookbook for Beginners

Discover the secrets to lose weight with Quick And Easy Mediterranean Recipes

Angela D. Lovato

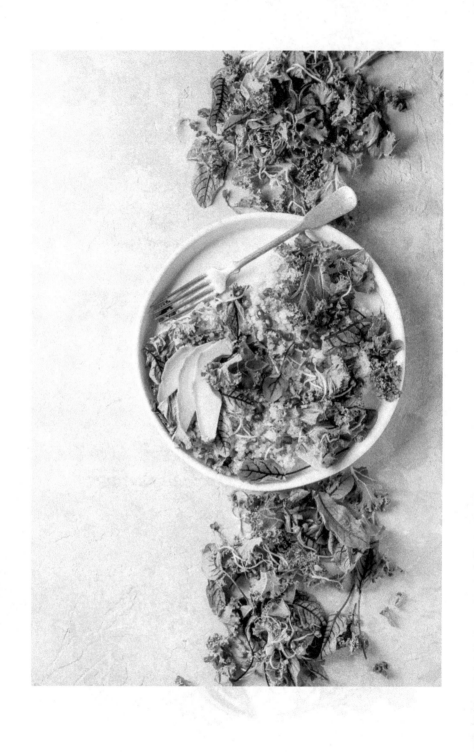

Table of content

MEDITERRANEAN BREAKFAST RECIPE

YOGURT CHEESE AND FRUIT

Serves 6

- 3 cups plain nonfat yogurt
- 1 teaspoon fresh lemon juice
- 1/2 cup orange juice
- 1/2 cup water
- 1 fresh Golden Delicious apple
- 1 fresh pear
- 1/4 cup honey
- 1/4 cup dried cranberries or raisins

Directions

- Prepare the yogurt cheese the day before by lining a colander or strainer with cheesecloth. Spoon the yogurt into the cheesecloth and place the strainer over a pot or bowl to catch the whey; refrigerate for at least 8 hours before serving.
- In a large mixing bowl, mix together the juices and water. Cut the apple and pear into wedges, and place the wedges in the juice mixture; let sit for at least 5 minutes. Strain off the liquid.
- When the yogurt is firm, remove from refrigerator, slice, and place on plates. Arrange the fruit wedges around the yogurt. Drizzle with honey and sprinkle with cranberries just before serving.

PANCETTA ON BAGUETTE

This Mediterranean version of "bacon and cheese" is incredibly delicious!

Serves 6

- 1 loaf baguette
- 1/2–1 teaspoon extra-virgin olive oil
- 6 ounces pancetta (ham, prosciutto, or Canadian bacon can be substituted)
- 1/4 cantaloupe, medium-diced
- 1/4 honeydew melon, medium-diced 3 ounces goat cheese
- Fresh-cracked black pepper, to taste

Directions

- Preheat the broiler on medium-high heat.
- Slice the baguette on the bias and place on baking sheet. Brush each slice with oil, then toast lightly on each side.
- Slice the pancetta paper-thin and into thin strips, then place on top of each baguette slice; place under broiler. Cook quickly, paying close attention so as not to burn (approximately 1 minute).
- While the baguette cooks, mix the cantaloupe and melon in a small bowl. When baguettes are done, remove them from the oven and place on a plate. To serve, sprinkle with cheese and black pepper. Garnish with a spoonful of melon mix.

VEGETABLE PITA WITH FETA CHEESE

Let your imagination go wild with seasonal veggies. This simple-to-prepare pita delight is delicious, and good for you, too.

Serves 6

- 1 eggplant, sliced into 1/2-inch pieces, lengthwise 1 zucchini, sliced into 1/2-inch pieces, lengthwise 1 yellow squash, sliced
- 1 red onion, cut into 1/3-inch rings
- 1 teaspoon virgin olive oil Fresh-cracked black pepper
- 6 whole-wheat pita bread
- 3 ounces feta cheese

Directions

- Preheat the oven to 375°F.
- Brush the sliced vegetables with oil and place on a racked baking sheet. Sprinkle with black pepper. Roast until tender. (The vegetables can be prepared the night before, refrigerated, then reheated or brought to room temperature before roasting.)
- Slice a 3-inch opening in the pitas to gain access to the pockets. Toast the pitas if desired. Fill the pitas with the cooked vegetables. Add cheese to each and serve.

ISRAELI COUSCOUS WITH DRIED-FRUIT CHUTNEY

Serves 6

- Chutney
- 1⁄4 cup medium-diced dried dates
- 1⁄4 cup medium-diced dried figs
- 1⁄4 cup medium-diced dried currants
- 1⁄4 cup slivered almonds Couscous
- 21⁄4 cups fresh orange juice
- 21⁄4 cups water
- 41⁄2 cups couscous
- 1 teaspoon grated orange rind
- 2 tablespoons nonfat plain yogurt

Directions

- Mix together all the chutney ingredients; set aside.
- Bring the orange juice and water to a boil in a medium-size pot. Stir in the couscous, then add the orange rind. Remove from heat immediately, cover, and let stand for 5 minutes. Fluff the mixture with a fork.
- Serve in bowls with a spoonful of chutney and a dollop of yogurt.

ALMOND MASCARPONE DUMPLINGS

Serves 6

- 1 cup whole-wheat flour
- 1 cup all-purpose unbleached flour
- ¼ cup ground almonds 4 egg whites
- 3 ounces mascarpone cheese
- 1 teaspoon extra-virgin olive oil
- 2 teaspoons apple juice
- 1 tablespoon butter
- ¼ cup honey

Directions

- Sift together both types of flour in a large bowl. Mix in the almonds. In a separate bowl, cream together the egg whites, cheese, oil, and juice on medium speed with an electric mixer.

- Combine the flour and egg white mixture with a dough hook on medium speed or by hand until a dough forms.

- Boil 1 gallon water in a medium-size saucepot. Take a spoonful of the dough and use a second spoon to push it into the boiling water. Cook until the dumpling floats to the top, about 5–10 minutes. You can cook several dumplings at once, just take care not to crowd the pot. Remove with a slotted spoon and drain on paper towels.

- Heat a medium-size sauté pan over medium-high heat. Add the butter, then place the dumplings in the pan and cook until light brown. Place on serving plates and drizzle with honey.

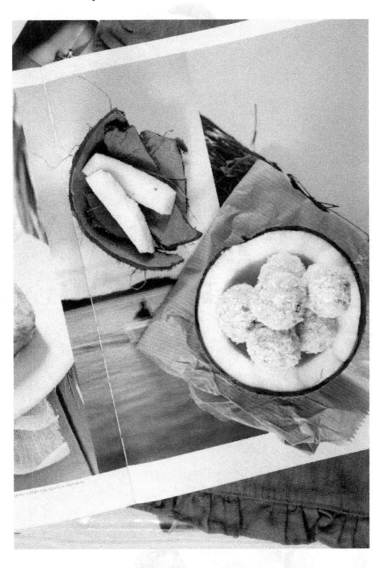

MEDITERRANEAN LUNCH RECIPE

Mediterranean chicken with roasted vegetables

Ingredients

- 250g baby new potatoes, thinly sliced
- 1 large courgette, diagonally sliced
- 1 red onion, cut into wedges
- 1 yellow pepper, seeded and cut into chunks
- 6 firm plum tomatoes, halved
- 12 black olives, pitted
- 2 skinless boneless chicken breast fillets, about 150g/5oz each
- 3 tbsp olive oil
- 1 rounded tbsp green pesto

Method

- Preheat the oven to 200C/ Gas 6/fan oven 180C. Spread the potatoes, courgette, onion, pepper and tomatoes in a shallow roasting tin and scatter over the olives. Season with salt and coarsely ground black pepper.
- Slash the flesh of each chicken breast 3-4 times using a sharp knife, then lay the chicken on top of the vegetables.
- Mix the olive oil and pesto together until well blended and spoon evenly over the chicken. Cover the tin with foil and cook for 30 minutes.
- Remove the foil from the tin. Return to the oven and cook for a further 10 minutes until the vegetables are juicy and

look tempting to eat and the chicken is cooked through (the juices should run clear when pierced with a skewer).

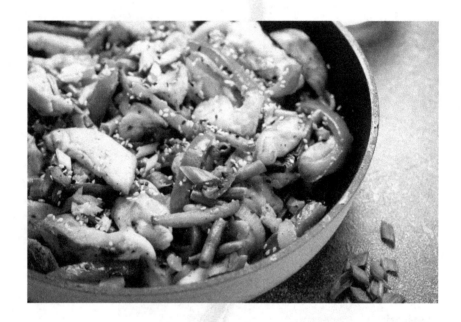

Roasted peppers with tomatoes & anchovies

Ingredients

- 4 red peppers , halved and deseeded
- 50g can anchovy in oil, drained
- 8 smallish tomatoes , halved
- 2 garlic cloves , thinly sliced
- 2 rosemary sprigs
- 2 tbsp olive oil

Method

- Heat oven to 160C/140C fan/gas 3. Put the peppers into a large baking dish, toss with a little of the oil from the anchovy can, then turn cut-side up. Roast for 40 mins, until soft but not collapsed.
- Slice 8 of the anchovies along their length. Put 2 halves of tomato, several garlic slices, a few little rosemary sprigs and two pieces of anchovy into the hollow of each pepper. Drizzle over the olive oil, then roast again for 30 mins until the tomatoes are soft and the peppers are filled with pools of tasty juice. Leave to cool and serve warm or at room temperature.

Mediterranean Stuffed Chicken Breasts

Ingredients

- ½ cup crumbled feta cheese
- ½ cup chopped roasted red bell peppers
- ½ cup chopped fresh spinach
- ¼ cup Kalamata olives, pitted and quartered
- 1 tablespoon chopped fresh basil
- 1 tablespoon chopped fresh flat-leaf parsley
- 2 cloves garlic, minced
- 4 (8 ounce) boneless, skinless chicken breasts
- ¼ teaspoon salt
- ½ teaspoon ground pepper
- 1 tablespoon extra-virgin olive oil
- 1 tablespoon lemon juice

Directions

- Preheat oven to 400 degrees F. Combine feta, roasted red peppers, spinach, olives, basil, parsley and garlic in a medium bowl.
- Using a small knife, cut a horizontal slit through the thickest portion of each chicken breast to form a pocket. Stuff each breast pocket with about 1/3 cup of the feta mixture; secure the pockets using wooden picks. Sprinkle the chicken evenly with salt and pepper.
- Heat oil in a large oven-safe skillet over medium-high heat. Arrange the stuffed breasts, top-sides down, in the pan; cook until golden, about 2 minutes. Carefully flip the

chicken; transfer the pan to the oven. Bake until an instant-read thermometer inserted in the thickest portion of the chicken registers 165 degrees F, 20 to 25 minutes. Drizzle the chicken evenly with lemon juice. Remove the wooden picks from the chicken before serving.

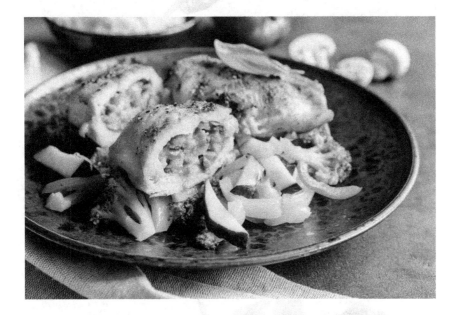

Charred Shrimp & Pesto Buddha Bowls

Ingredients

- ⅓ cup prepared pesto
- 2 tablespoons balsamic vinegar
- 1 tablespoon extra-virgin olive oil
- ½ teaspoon salt
- ¼ teaspoon ground pepper
- 1 pound peeled and deveined large shrimp (16-20 count), patted dry
- 4 cups arugula
- 2 cups cooked quinoa
- 1 cup halved cherry tomatoes
- 1 avocado, diced

Directions

- Whisk pesto, vinegar, oil, salt and pepper in a large bowl. Remove 4 tablespoons of the mixture to a small bowl; set both bowls aside.
- Heat a large cast-iron skillet over medium-high heat. Add shrimp and cook, stirring, until just cooked through with a slight char, 4 to 5 minutes. Remove to a plate.
- Add arugula and quinoa to the large bowl with the vinaigrette and toss to coat. Divide the arugula mixture between 4 bowls. Top with tomatoes, avocado and shrimp. Drizzle each bowl with 1 tablespoon of the reserved pesto mixture.

Sheet-Pan Salmon with Sweet Potatoes & Broccoli

Ingredients

- 3 tablespoons low-fat mayonnaise
- 1 teaspoon chili powder
- 2 medium sweet potatoes, peeled and cut into 1-inch cubes
- 4 teaspoons olive oil, divided
- ½ teaspoon salt, divided
- ¼ teaspoon ground pepper, divided
- 4 cups broccoli florets (8 oz.; 1 medium crown)
- 1 ¼ pounds salmon fillet, cut into 4 portions
- 2 limes, 1 zested and juiced, 1 cut into wedges for serving
- ¼ cup crumbled feta or cotija cheese
- ½ cup chopped fresh cilantro

Directions

- Preheat oven to 425 degrees F. Line a large rimmed baking sheet with foil and coat with cooking spray.
- Combine mayonnaise and chili powder in a small bowl. Set aside.
- Toss sweet potatoes with 2 tsp. oil, 1/4 tsp. salt, and 1/8 tsp. pepper in a medium bowl. Spread on the prepared baking sheet. Roast for 15 minutes.
- Meanwhile, toss broccoli with the remaining 2 tsp. oil, 1/4 tsp. salt, and 1/8 tsp. pepper in the same bowl. Remove the baking sheet from oven. Stir the sweet potatoes and

move them to the sides of the pan. Arrange salmon in the center of the pan and spread the broccoli on either side, among the sweet potatoes. Spread 2 Tbsp. of the mayonnaise mixture over the salmon. Bake until the sweet potatoes are tender and the salmon flakes easily with a fork, about 15 minutes.

- Meanwhile, add lime zest and lime juice to the remaining 1 Tbsp. mayonnaise; mix well.
- Divide the salmon among 4 plates and top with cheese and cilantro. Divide the sweet potatoes and broccoli among the plates and drizzle with the lime-mayonnaise sauce. Serve with lime wedges and any remaining sauce.

Mediterranean Ravioli with Artichokes & Olives

Ingredients

- 2 (8 ounce) packages frozen or refrigerated spinach-and-ricotta ravioli
- ½ cup oil-packed sun-dried tomatoes, drained (2 tablespoons oil reserved)
- 1 (10 ounce) package frozen quartered artichoke hearts, thawed
- 1 (15 ounce) can no-salt-added cannellini beans, rinsed
- ¼ cup Kalamata olives, sliced
- 3 tablespoons toasted pine nuts
- ¼ cup chopped fresh basil

Directions

- Bring a large pot of water to a boil. Cook ravioli according to package directions. Drain and toss with 1 tablespoon reserved oil; set aside.
- Heat the remaining 1 tablespoon oil in a large nonstick skillet over medium heat. Add artichokes and beans; sauté until heated through, 2 to 3 minutes.
- Fold in the cooked ravioli, sun-dried tomatoes, olives, pine nuts and basil.

MEDITERRANEAN SALAD RECIPES

KALAMATA OLIVE DRESSING

Serves 4

- 1⁄4 cup chopped red onions
- 1 clove garlic, peeled and smashed
- 1⁄2 cup pitted kalamata olives
- 2 sun-dried tomatoes, packed in olive oil, rinsed and chopped
- 1⁄2 teaspoon dried oregano
- 2 tablespoons red wine vinegar
- 1 tablespoon balsamic vinegar
- 1 teaspoon Dijon mustard
- 1⁄2 teaspoon pepper
- 2⁄3 cup extra-virgin olive oil

Directions

- Add all the ingredients to a food processor, and process until they are well incorporated.
- Refrigerate the dressing until it is needed.

CUCUMBER AND DILL DRESSING

This dressing pairs wonderfully with salad greens, ripe tomatoes, and some peppery radish slices.

Serves 4

- 1⁄2 medium English cucumber, grated
- 3⁄4 teaspoon salt, divided
- 1⁄2 cup strained Greek yogurt
- 1⁄4 cup whole milk
- 2 tablespoons mayonnaise
- 2 teaspoons fresh lemon juice
- 1 scallion (white part only), ends trimmed and thinly sliced
- 1 clove garlic, peeled and minced
- 2 tablespoons chopped fresh dill
- 1⁄4 teaspoon pepper

Directions

- Place cucumber and 1⁄4 teaspoon salt in a fine-mesh strainer over a medium bowl. Strain for 30 minutes. Squeeze any remaining water from the cucumber.
- Combine the cucumber and remaining ingredients in a medium bowl. Stir well to incorporate the ingredients.
- Adjust the seasoning if necessary. Refrigerate the dressing in a tight jar for up to 1 week.

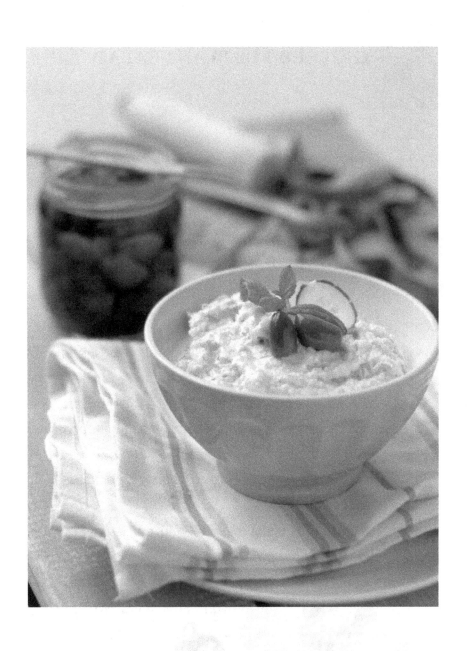

27

GRILLED EGGPLANT SALAD

Serves 4

- 1 large eggplant
- 2 tablespoons salt, plus more to taste
- 2 or 3 tomatoes
- Small bunch of parsley, finely chopped
- 2 cloves garlic, pressed or very finely diced Pepper to taste
- 1 tablespoon dried oregano
- 1/4 cup extra-virgin olive oil

Directions

- Slice eggplant into discs along length—not too thin and not too thick, about 1/4 inch thickness is ideal. Fill a large mixing bowl or pot with water, add 2 tablespoons of salt, and mix well; place eggplant discs in salt bath and set a plate over the top to weigh them down. Soak for 20–30 minutes. Mix periodically to ensure salty water soaks them completely.
- Dice tomatoes; place in bowl. Add parsley, garlic, salt, pepper, oregano, and 2–3 tablespoons olive oil; mix well and set aside.
- Light a grill and set on high temperature. When grilling surface is ready, spray or wipe with vegetable oil.
- Using your hands and working quickly over the grill, brush (or spray) downward-facing side of each slice of eggplant with a little olive oil; place across grill, starting from the top left rear section and filling the entire surface in rows. Once

all the eggplant discs are on the grill, give the upward-facing sides a brush (or spray) of olive oil. Grill until visibly softened around the edges and centers, approximately 6–8 minutes. Allow each side a few minutes to cook through and absorb oil, but watch them carefully.

- Brush with olive oil again; turn over. Grill another few minutes; give final brushing of oil. Leave on grill another minute or so; remove onto platter or dish.
- Arrange several eggplant discs on a serving plate, top with chopped tomato mixture, sprinkle with oregano, and serve with crusty bread.

MEDITERRANEAN POULTRY RECIPES

CHICKEN WITH YOGURT

Serves 4

- 1 whole chicken
- 2 lemons, halved
- Salt and pepper
- 2 cups strained yogurt
- 2 tablespoons milk
- 2 tablespoons fresh mint, chopped
- 2 cups dry bread crumbs
- 1/2 cup salted butter

Directions

- Preheat the oven to 350°F.
- Wash chicken well inside and out and pat dry with a paper towel. Cut chicken into sections; rub vigorously with lemon halves and sprinkle with salt and pepper. Place pieces in a colander; let stand for 1 hour.
- Place yogurt in a mixing bowl. Add milk and mint; mix well with a whisk until smooth.
- Dip each piece of chicken into yogurt mix, then cover entirely with a good sprinkling of bread crumbs. Place on a greased roasting pan; drizzle melted butter over the top.
- Bake for about 1 hour, until the chicken pieces are golden brown.
- Serve with a side of rice or fried potatoes.

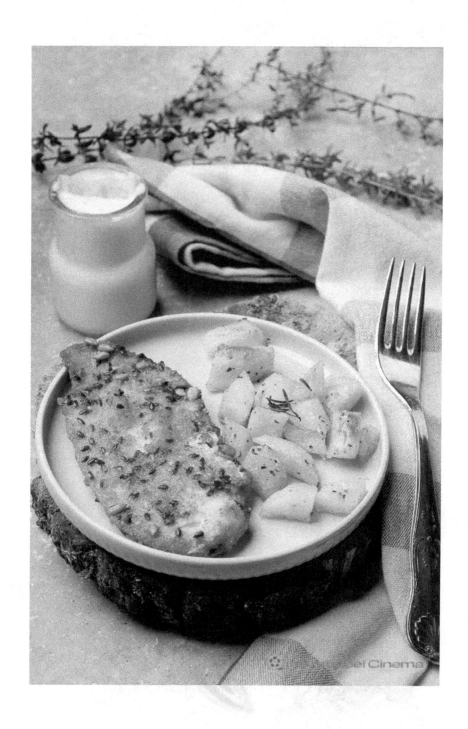

CHICKEN WITH EGG NOODLES AND WALNUTS

Serves 4–6

- 1 whole chicken
- 1/2 cup extra-virgin olive oil 1 onion, diced
- 1/4 cup butter 2 cups tomato pulp, minced and sieved
- 4 cups boiling water
- 1 tablespoon fresh mint, chopped
- Salt and pepper
- 1 pound square egg noodles (Greek hilopites)
- 1/2 cup crushed walnuts Grated myzithra or Parmesan cheese for garnish (optional)

Directions

- Wash chicken well inside and out and pat dry with a paper towel. Cut into sections.
- Heat oil. Sauté onion slightly; add butter and chicken and sauté thoroughly on all sides.
- Add tomatoes, boiling water, mint, salt, and pepper. Bring to a boil; cover and simmer over medium-low heat for 30 minutes.
- Add egg noodles and crushed walnuts; give a good stir. Cover and continue to simmer for another 30 minutes.
- Stir before serving hot with some grated myzithra or Parmesan cheese over each helping.

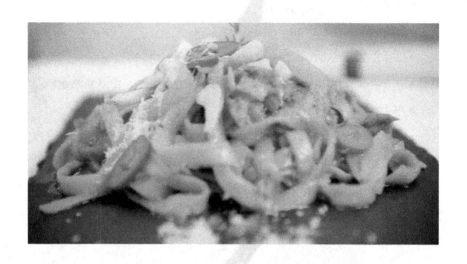

STUFFED GRILLED CHICKEN BREASTS

Serves 6

- 6 large boneless, skinless chicken breasts
- 1 cup crumbled Greek feta cheese
- 1/2 cup finely minced sun-dried tomatoes
- 1 teaspoon dried oregano
- 2 tablespoons extra-virgin olive oil
- Salt and pepper

Directions

- Wash chicken breasts well and pat dry with a paper towel.
- In a bowl, mix feta with sun-dried tomatoes and oregano; combine thoroughly.
- Place each chicken breast on a flat surface; using a sharp paring knife, carefully slit the top edge of each breast and make a deep incision that runs within the length of each breast. Be careful not to pierce any holes that would allow stuffing to seep out while grilling.
- Use a small spoon to stuff an equal portion of cheese mixture into each breast; use poultry pins or toothpicks to close openings.
- Sear breasts in a heated frying pan with olive oil, approximately 2–3 minutes per side.
- Sprinkle with salt and pepper; cook on a prepared grill over high heat for about 15 minutes, approximately 8 minutes per side. Serve immediately.

CHICKEN LIVERS IN RED WINE

Serves 4

- 1 pound chicken livers
- 1 cup chicken broth
- 1/2 cup butter 1 small onion, diced
- 1 tablespoon all-purpose flour
- 1/2 cup red wine Salt and pepper
- 2 tablespoons fresh parsley, finely chopped

Directions

- Wash chicken livers thoroughly and drain well before using. Bring broth to a boil in a small pan and let simmer over low heat.
- Melt butter in another frying pan. Slightly sauté onion; add chicken livers and cook over high heat for 3–5 minutes, stirring constantly to avoid browning.
- Sprinkle flour over top of livers and butter; continue to stir well to form a sauce in the bottom of the pan. Stir constantly to avoid clumping.
- Slowly add hot broth to the pan with the livers, stirring constantly. Turn heat to high and slowly add wine; continue to simmer and stir several minutes. Reduce heat to low; cook for another 5–10 minutes to thicken sauce.
- Season with salt and pepper and serve hot with chopped parsley as a garnish over a bed of mashed potatoes.

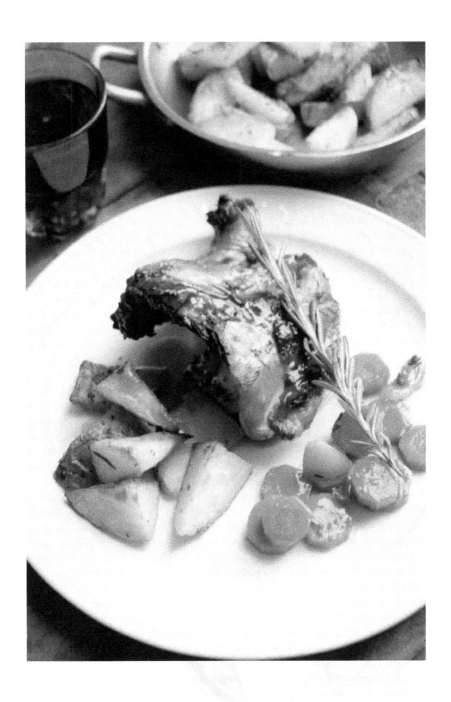

MEDITERRANEAN
SEAFOOD RECIPES

GRILLED SEA BASS

Serves 4

- 4 whole sea bass (1 1⁄2 pounds each), gutted and scaled
  Salt and pepper
- 4 lemons
- 1⁄4 cup extra-virgin olive oil
- 1 teaspoon dried oregano
- 1 cup fresh parsley, finely chopped

Directions

- Wash the fish well inside and out. Using a sharp knife, cut several diagonal slits on both sides of each fish. Sprinkle with salt and pepper, including inside cavity, and set aside.
- Squeeze juice from 2 lemons and mix with olive oil and oregano.
- Slice remaining 2 lemons into thin slices and stuff each fish with chopped parsley and several lemon slices.
- Brush both sides of each fish liberally with olive oil and lemon mixture and set aside for 10 minutes.
- Heat grill to medium heat; brush grilling rack with oil. Place fish on hot rack and close grill cover.
- Cook for 15 minutes, until fish flakes easily. Brush with remaining olive oil and lemon mixture and serve hot.

OCTOPUS IN WINE

Serves 4

- 1 large octopus
- 1 tablespoon white vinegar
- 1/2 cup extra-virgin olive oil
- 3 onions, sliced
- 4 tomatoes, diced and sieved (fresh or canned)
- 1 cup white wine
- 2 bay leaves
- 1 teaspoon whole peppercorns
- Salt and pepper
- 1/2 cup drained capers
- 1/4 cup water

Directions

- Place octopus in a saucepan with vinegar; cover and simmer over low heat until soft, approximately 15–20 minutes. Remove and cut into small pieces.
- Heat olive oil in a frying pan and sauté onions until soft.
- Add tomatoes, wine, bay leaves, peppercorns, salt, and pepper; simmer for 15 minutes.
- Add octopus, capers, and water; simmer until sauce has thickened. Remove the bay leaves; serve hot.

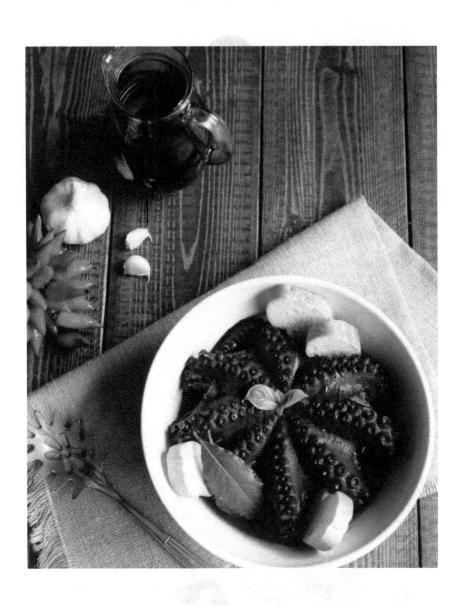

CIOPPINO

Serves 6

- clams
- mussels
- ounces skinless, boneless cod fillet
- 1 shallot
- 1 yellow onion
- 2 cloves garlic
- 2 stalks celery
- 2 carrots
- 3 plum tomatoes
- 1 cup dry white wine
- 3 cups Fish Stock
- 1⁄2 teaspoon saffron threads
- 1⁄4 teaspoon dried red pepper flakes
- 1⁄2 teaspoon extra-virgin olive oil
- 1⁄4 teaspoon capers

Directions

- Rinse the clams in ice-cold water. Thoroughly clean the mussels. Cut the cod into chunks. Small-dice the shallot, onion, garlic, and celery. Peel and small-dice the carrots and tomatoes (see Tomato Fritters recipe in Chapter 4 for tomato peeling instructions).

- Place the cod, vegetables, wine, stock, saffron, and pepper flakes into a large stockpot; simmer over medium heat for approximately 1 hour.
- Add the shellfish and cook until the shells open. (Discard any clams or mussels that do not open!)
- Ladle the Cioppino into bowls. Drizzle with the oil and sprinkle with the

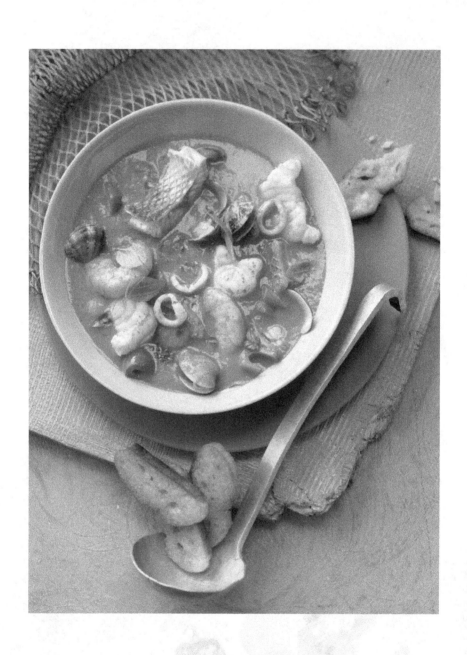

STEAMED SNOW CRAB LEGS

Serves 6

- 6 snow crab claw clusters
- 2 pounds parsnips
- 6 celery stalks
- 1 yellow onion
- 1/2 bunch fresh parsley
- 1/2 cup white wine (Pinot Grigio or Sauvignon Blanc) Juice of 1 lemon
- 1 cup Fish Stock
- 3 bay leaves Fresh-cracked black pepper, to taste

Directions

- Clean the crab legs thoroughly in ice-cold water. Peel and roughly chop the parsnips. Roughly chop the celery and onion. Chop the parsley.
- Combine all the ingredients except the snow crab in a medium-size saucepot and bring to a boil; reduce to a simmer and cook uncovered for approximately 20–30 minutes.
- Add the crab legs, and cook for 10–15 minutes, until the crab is cooked. Remove the bay leaves, then serve.

MEDITERRANEAN MEAT, BEEF AND PORK RECIPES

ZUCCHINI STUFFED WITH MEAT AND RICE

Serves 6

- 1⁄4 cup extra-virgin olive oil 2 medium onions, peeled and finely diced
- 3 cloves garlic, peeled and minced
- 1 1⁄2 cups chopped fresh parsley 3⁄4 cup chopped fresh dill 1⁄2 cup chopped fresh mint 2⁄3 cup tomato sauce
- 1⁄4 cup plus 2 tablespoons water plus 3 cups hot water, divided
- 1 1⁄2 cups Arborio rice 2 pounds extra-lean ground beef
- 1 tablespoon salt
- 3⁄4 teaspoon black pepper 10 medium zucchini, peeled, cut in half, and cored
- 4 tablespoons all-purpose flour
- 3 large eggs
- 6 tablespoons fresh lemon juice

Directions

- Preheat the oven to 375°F. Heat the oil in a large skillet over medium-high heat for 30 seconds. Reduce the heat to medium and add the onions and garlic. Cook for 5–6 minutes or until the onions soften. Stir in the parsley, dill, and mint. Add the tomato sauce, 1⁄4 cup of water, and the rice. Cook for 10 minutes while stirring. Stir in the beef, salt, and pepper. Take the skillet off the heat.

- Stuff the zucchini with the filling. Place them in a roasting pan big enough to hold them in a single layer. Pour 3 cups of hot water into the roasting pan, cover it with a lid, and bake for 60 minutes. Carefully tilt the roasting pan and pour any remaining liquid from the pan into a bowl.
- Reserve the liquid and the zucchini.
- In a large bowl, whisk the flour and 2 tablespoons of water to form a slurry. Whisk in the eggs and lemon juice. Continuing to whisk vigorously, slowly add a ladle of the reserved liquid into the egg-lemon mixture. Continue whisking and slowly add another 2 ladles (one at a time) into the egg-lemon mixture. Adjust the seasoning with salt, if necessary.
- Pour the avgolemono over the zucchini and shake the pan to allow the sauce to blend in. Let it cool for 15 minutes before serving warm.

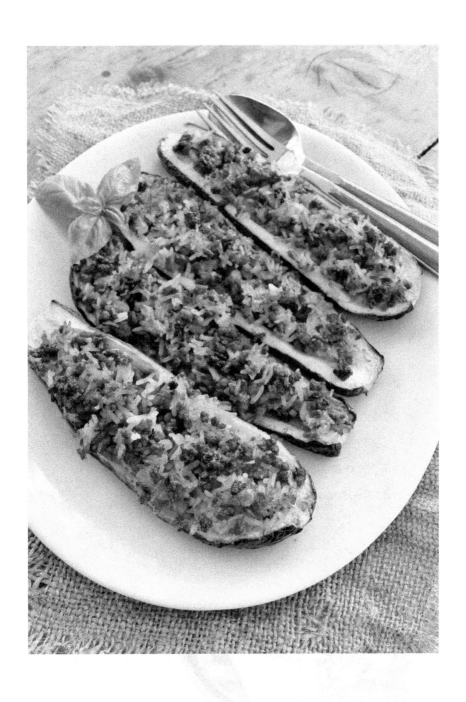

49

GREEK-STYLE FLANK STEAK

Serves 4

- 1/4 cup extra-virgin olive oil 7 or 8 cloves garlic, peeled and smashed
- 4 or 5 chopped scallions, ends trimmed
- 1 tablespoon Dijon mustard
- 1/3 cup balsamic vinegar 2 bay leaves
- 2 tablespoons fresh thyme leaves
- 2 tablespoons fresh rosemary leaves
- 1 teaspoon dried oregano
- 1 1/2 teaspoons salt, divided 3/4 teaspoon pepper, divided 1 (2-pound) large flank steak
- 3 tablespoons vegetable oil

Directions

- In a food processor, process the olive oil, garlic, scallions, mustard, vinegar, bay leaves, thyme, rosemary, oregano, 1 teaspoon salt, and 1/2 teaspoon pepper. Thoroughly incorporate the ingredients in the marinade.

- Rub the steak with the marinade and place in a medium baking dish. Cover and refrigerate for 3 hours. Return the steak to room temperature before grilling. Wipe most of the marinade off the steak and season with remaining salt and pepper.
- Preheat a gas or charcoal grill to medium-high. Brush the grill surface to make sure it is thoroughly clean. When the grill is ready, dip a clean tea towel in the vegetable oil and wipe the grill surface with the oil. Place the meat on the grill and grill for 4 minutes a side.
- Let the steak rest for 5 minutes before serving.

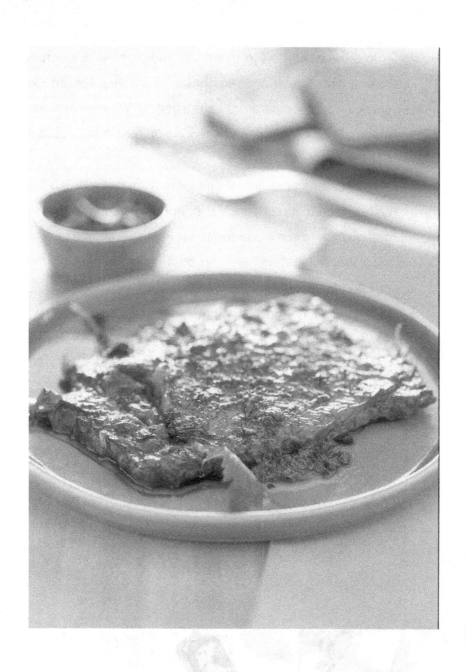

CHEESE-STUFFED BIFTEKI

Serves 6

- 2 pounds medium ground beef
- 2 medium onions, peeled and grated
- 3 slices of bread, soaked in water, hand squeezed, and crumbled
- 1 tablespoon minced garlic
- 1 teaspoon dried oregano
- 1 teaspoon chopped fresh parsley
- 1⁄4 teaspoon ground allspice 2 tablespoons salt
- 1 teaspoon pepper
- 6 (1-inch) cubes Graviera cheese
- 3 tablespoons vegetable oil

Directions

- In a large bowl, combine all the ingredients (except the cheese and vegetable oil) and mix thoroughly.
- Using your hands, form twelve (4" × 1⁄2") patties with the meat. Place the patties on a tray, cover them with plastic wrap, and refrigerate for 4 hours or overnight. Allow the patties to come to room temperature before grilling.
- Take a piece of cheese and place it on the middle of a patty. Place another patty on top and press them together to form one burger. Using your fingers, pinch the entire perimeter of the burger so that when you grill, the burger will hold together and the cheese will not leak out.

- Preheat a gas or charcoal grill to medium-high. Brush the grill surface to make sure it is thoroughly clean. When the grill is ready, dip a clean tea towel in the vegetable oil and wipe the grill surface with the oil. Place the burgers on the grill and grill for 5 minutes a side.
- Allow the burgers to rest for 5 minutes before serving.

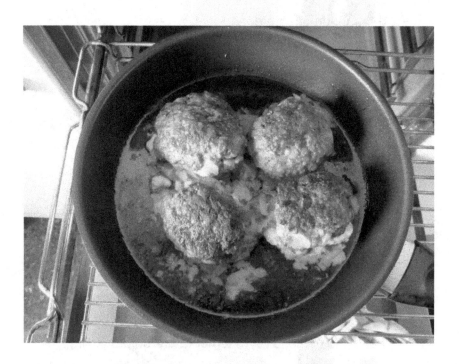

MEATBALLS IN EGG-LEMON SAUCE

Serves 6

- 2 pounds lean ground veal
- 2 medium onions, finely diced
- 1/2 cup dry bread crumbs 1 egg, beaten, plus 2 eggs
- 1/4 cup extra-virgin olive oil, divided
- 1/4 cup fresh mint, finely chopped
- 1/4 cup fresh parsley, finely chopped
- 1 teaspoon dried oregano
- Salt and pepper to taste
- 4 cups Beef Stock or Veal Stock Juice of 1 lemon

Directions

- Preheat the oven to 400°F.
- In a large mixing bowl, combine meat, onions, bread crumbs, 1 beaten egg, 2 tablespoons olive oil, mint, parsley, oregano, salt, and pepper; mix together well with your hands.
- Using your fingers, take up small pieces of meat mix and fashion into meatballs about the size of a golf ball. Place in rows in a baking dish greased with the remaining olive oil. Bake for 30–40 minutes, until cooked.
- In a stockpot, bring stock to a boil. Add the meatballs; cover and simmer for 10 minutes.
- Beat the 2 remaining eggs in a mixing bowl; slowly add lemon juice and some of the hot stock in slow streams as you beat them to achieve a frothy mix.

- Pour egg-lemon mix into the pot with the meatballs. Cover and simmer for another 2–3 minutes and serve immediately.

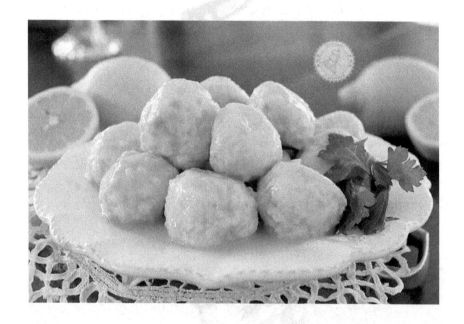

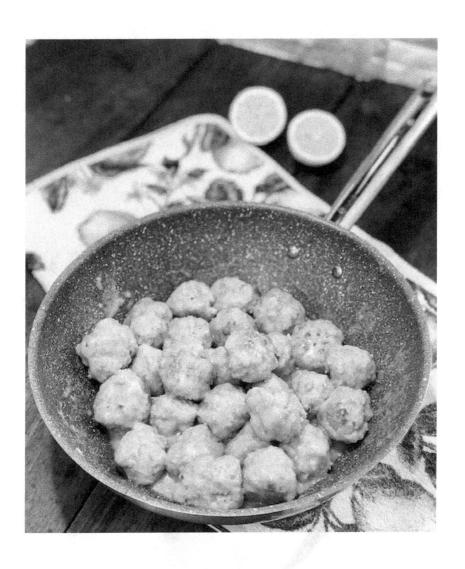

VEGETARIAN AND LEGUMES MEDITERRANEAN RECIPES

CHICKPEA RISSOLES

Serves 4

- 1 pound chickpeas (soaked overnight if dry)
- egg
- 1 tablespoon dried oregano or finely chopped fresh
- 3 tablespoons finely chopped fresh mint
- 3 tablespoons flour
- 1 teaspoon pepper
- 1⁄2 teaspoon salt
- 3 tablespoons bread crumbs Vegetable oil for deep-frying

Directions

- Boil chickpeas for 30 minutes, or until soft; drain and purée with egg, oregano, mint, flour, pepper, and salt.
- Scrape chickpea purée into a mixing bowl. Add bread crumbs; mix well.
- Spread a sheet of wax paper on the counter/cutting board. Spoon about 1⁄3 of the chickpea mixture in an even line along the horizontal center of the wax paper. Fold over the bottom half of wax paper and, using the flat of your hand, roll mixture into a long cylindrical shape (similar to using a sushi roller). Cut resulting cylindrical shape into 3 equal pieces or "sausages." Repeat to use up the rest of the chickpea mixture.
- Place rissoles into sizzling oil; fry for 5–6 minutes, making sure to turn often if the oil does not completely cover the

rissoles. Remove with a slotted spoon; set on paper towels a few minutes to drain.

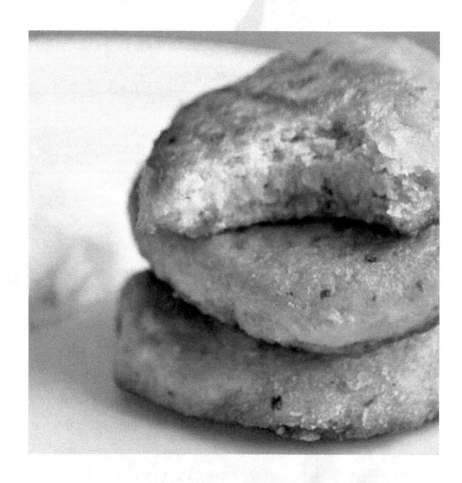

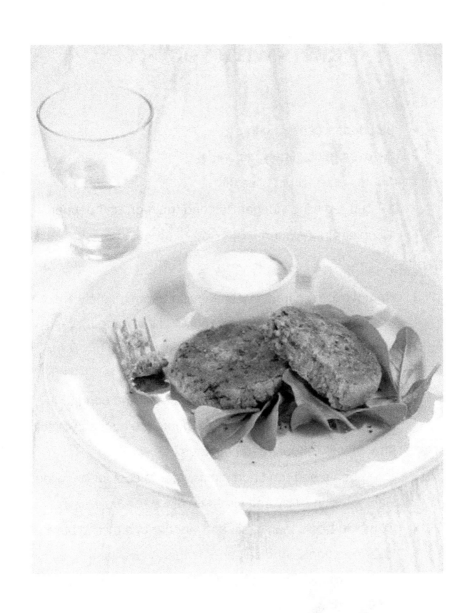

BEETS WITH YOGURT

Serves 2–4

- 2 pounds fresh red beets
- 3 cloves garlic, finely minced
- 1⁄4 cup extra-virgin olive oil
- 1⁄4 cup red wine vinegar Salt and fresh-ground pepper
- 1 cup strained yogurt

Directions

- Remove leaves from beets, leaving approximately 1 inch of stem along with the lower root, if still attached. Wash beets gently in cold water, making sure not to break the skin.
- Place beets in a pot of cold water; cover and bring to a boil. Cook on medium heat until beets are cooked yet still firm, usually about 45–50 minutes.
- Drain beets and run under cold water to cool for handling. Peel the skin away and slice into discs.
- Combine beets, garlic, oil, and vinegar in a mixing bowl; toss thoroughly. Add salt and pepper. Cover and refrigerate for 2 hours. Serve with a good dollop of yogurt on the side.

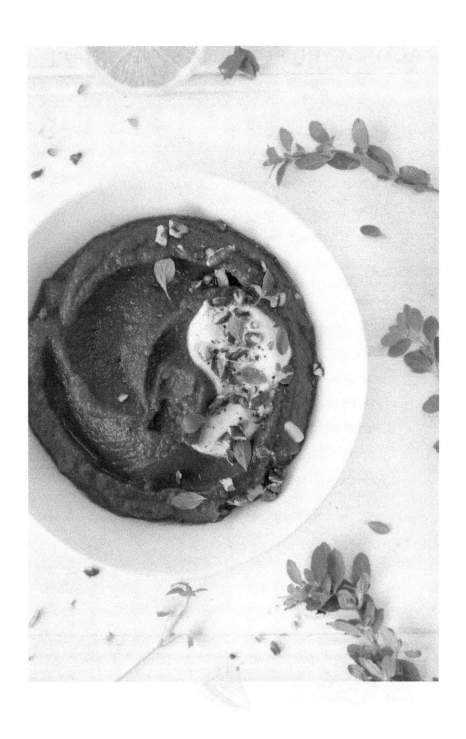

BLACK-EYED PEAS AND SWISS CHARD

Serves 4

- 1 cup dry black-eyed peas
- 1⁄4 cup extra-virgin olive oil
- 1 teaspoon dried oregano Salt and pepper
- 2 pounds Swiss chard
- Juice of 1 lemon

Directions

- Soak peas overnight. Drain and rinse before using.
- Bring a pot of water to boil; simmer peas for 15 minutes.
- Drain water from the pot. Add fresh water, olive oil, oregano, and salt and pepper; bring to a boil again. Simmer on medium-low heat for 30 minutes.
- Chop Swiss chard leaves into ribbons; add to the pot after 30 minutes. Simmer for another 5 minutes.
- Sprinkle with lemon juice. Serve warm or cold.

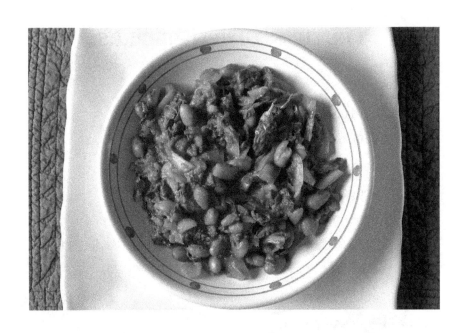

LENTIL-STUFFED PEPPERS

Serves 6

- 2 medium yellow onions
- 2 stalks celery
- 2 carrots
- 6 sprigs oregano
- 1 tablespoon olive oil
- 1 cup Basic Vegetable Stock plus 3 cups, divided 3 cups red lentils
- 6 bell peppers
- 3 ounces feta cheese
- Fresh-cracked black pepper, to taste

Directions

- Finely dice the onions and celery. Peel and finely dice the carrots. Reserve the top parts of the oregano sprigs and chop the remaining leaves.
- Heat the oil over medium heat in a large saucepot. Add the onions, carrots, and celery; sauté for 5 minutes, then add 1 cup Basic Vegetable Stock and the lentils. Simmer for 15–20 minutes, until the lentils are fully cooked.
- Cut off the tops of the peppers, leaving the stems attached, and remove the seeds. Place the peppers in a shallow pot with the 3 cups Basic Vegetable Stock. Cover and simmer for 10 minutes, then remove from heat.
- In a bowl, mix together the lentil mixture, the chopped oregano, feta, and black pepper; spoon the mixture into

the peppers. Serve the peppers with the stem tops ajar. Garnish with reserved oregano tops.

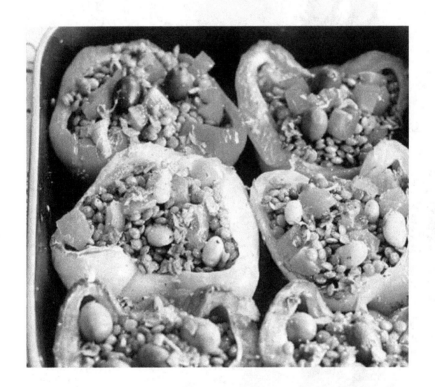

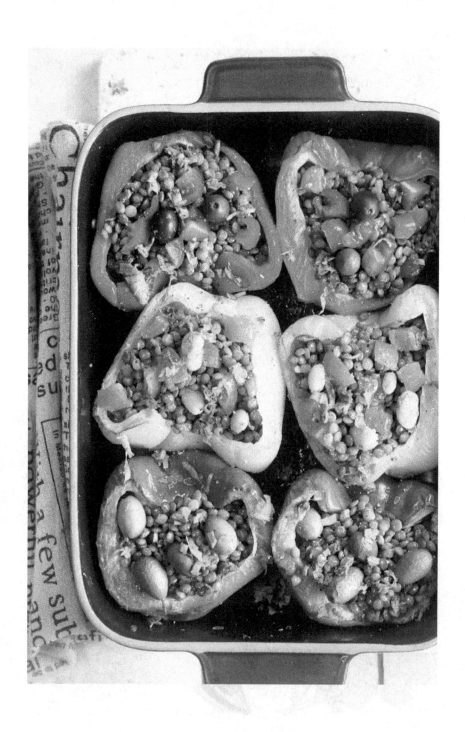

MEDITERRANEAN DESSERTS

SAUTÉED STRAWBERRIES IN YOGURT SOUP

To make the most of this delectable dessert, serve with a dollop of nonfat vanilla yogurt.

Serves 6

- 1 cup skim milk
- 1 vanilla bean
- 2 tablespoons granulated sugar
- 2 cups nonfat plain yogurt
- 1 pint strawberries
- 1 tablespoon unsalted butter
- 1/4 cup brown sugar

Directions

- Heat the milk with the vanilla bean and granulated sugar in a small saucepan; let cool and remove vanilla bean. When the milk is completely cooled, whisk in the yogurt.
- Slice the strawberries. Melt the butter and toss with the strawberries.
- Serve the yogurt soup in a shallow bowl. Dollop with the strawberry mixture and sprinkle with brown sugar.

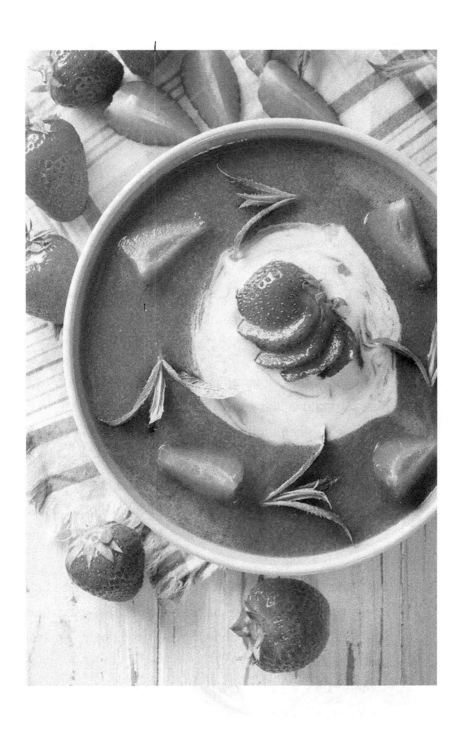

CITRUS SHERBET

Serves 8

- 4 Valencia oranges
- 2 Ruby Red grapefruits
- 1 key lime
- 1¼ cups granulated sugar ⅓ cup water 3 egg whites
- ¼ teaspoon cream of tartar
- ¼ teaspoon salt Edible orchid or mint leaves, for garnish Juice the oranges, grapefruits, and lime, then measure out 3 cups of unfiltered juice and set aside.

Directions

- In a saucepan, combine the sugar and water. Bring to a boil, stirring until the sugar dissolves. Cook to 238°F (soft ball on a candy thermometer).
- While this is cooking, beat the egg whites with the cream of tartar and salt until stiff. Slowly pour the hot syrup into the mixing bowl with the egg whites, continuing to beat at high speed. Continue to beat until the mixture is stiff and glossy (approximately 5 minutes).
- Stir in the juices, then pour into a shallow pan. Freeze until almost firm, then return to the bowl. Beat again until blended. Return to the container for scooping or smaller serving dish and freeze.
- To serve, remove from freezer, allowing 15 minutes before serving. Scoop and garnish.

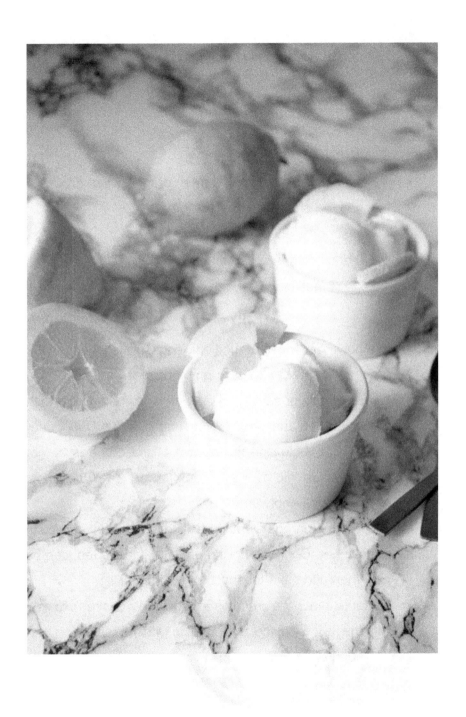

ORANGE CREPES

Serves 6

- 1⁄2 cup flour 2 whole eggs
- 2 egg whites
- 1⁄2 cup skim milk 11⁄2 cups fresh orange juice, divided 1 teaspoon fresh orange zest, divided
- 1⁄2 teaspoon melted butter
- 1 teaspoon cold unsalted butter
- 1⁄4 cup confectioners' sugar

Directions

- In a bowl, mix together the flour, eggs, milk, 1⁄4 cup of the orange juice, and 1⁄2 teaspoon of the orange zest.
- Heat a griddle or sauté pan over medium heat. Brush with melted butter and pour in the batter. When the batter begins to bubble and the bottom of the crepe is a light golden brown, flip over and cook for just a few seconds. Remove and keep warm.
- Prepare the orange syrup by boiling the remaining juice in a small pot. Continue boiling until the juice is reduced by half, then add the 1 teaspoon of cold butter.
- To serve, place the crepe on a plate (fold if desired), drizzle with the reduced juice, and sprinkle with the remaining zest and sugar.

CLAFOUTIS WITH FRUIT

Serves 2

- 2 teaspoons unsalted butter, divided
- 2 cups seasonal fruit (cherries, raspberries, blueberries, blackberries, etc.)
- 1/2 cup granulated sugar, divided 2 eggs
- 11/2 cups milk 6 teaspoons all-purpose flour Confectioners' sugar

Directions

- Preheat the oven to 400°F.
- Butter individual ovenproof dishes using 1 teaspoon of butter. Sprinkle the fruit with 1/4 cup of the granulated sugar and arrange in the bottom of each dish.
- Mix together the eggs, milk, remaining butter and granulated sugar, and the flour 1 teaspoon at a time until a smooth batter is formed.
- Pour this mixture over the fruit and bake for approximately 20 minutes, then reduce heat to 325°F and bake 10 minutes more. Insert a knife in the custard to test doneness. If the custard sticks to the knife, it isn't done yet. When the knife comes out clean, then it is done.
- Sprinkle with confectioners' sugar and serve.

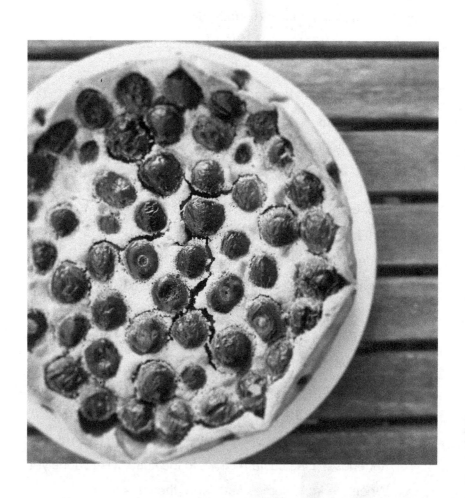

MEDITERRANEAN BREAD

SMOKED EGGPLANT AND FETA PIE FILLING

Serves 12

- 4 large eggplants, skins pierced several times with a fork
- 1 teaspoon red wine vinegar
- 2 cups crumbled feta cheese
- 4 large eggs, beaten
- 1/2 teaspoon pepper

Directions

- Preheat a gas or charcoal grill to medium-high. Grill the eggplants for 20–30 minutes or until the skin is completely charred and the insides are soft. Cool for 10 minutes. Cut them open lengthwise and scoop out the softened flesh, discarding the charred skin.
- In a large bowl, combine the eggplant and vinegar. Stir in feta, eggs, and pepper. The filling can be used immediately, or it can be refrigerated. If you refrigerate the filling, bring it to room temperature before using it.

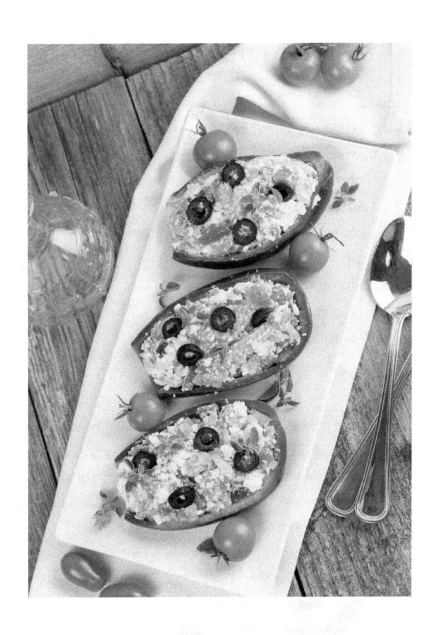

LEEK AND CHEESE PIE FILLING

Serves 12

- 1⁄4 cup extra-virgin olive oil 4 leeks (white parts only), ends trimmed, thoroughly cleaned, cut lengthwise, and finely chopped 2 medium zucchini, peeled and grated
- 1 teaspoon salt
- 1 cup ricotta cheese
- 1 cup crumbled feta cheese
- 3 large eggs, beaten
- 1⁄2 cup chopped fresh dill
- 1⁄2 teaspoon pepper

Directions:

- Heat the oil in a large skillet over medium heat. Add the leeks and cook for 5 minutes or until they soften. Stir in zucchini and salt. Reduce heat to medium-low and cook for 30 minutes. Take the skillet off the heat and cool the mixture to room temperature.
- In a large bowl, combine the leek mixture, ricotta, feta, eggs, dill, and pepper. The filling can be used immediately, or it can be refrigerated. If you refrigerate the filling, bring it to room temperature before using it.

MEDITERRANEAN RICE AND GRAINS

Healthy Butternut Squash Grain Bowl

Ingredients

- 1 cup butternut squash cubes
- 1 teaspoon olive oil
- 1 teaspoon maple syrup
- 1/4 teaspoon cinnamon
- 1/4 teaspoon freshly cracked pepper
- Pinch salt
- 1/4 cup pecans
- 1 cup cooked wild rice
- 2 cups baby spinach or spring mix
- 1 small Honeycrisp apple
- 1/4 cup dried cranberries

Preparation

- Heat oven to 400F. Line a baking sheet with parchment or a silicone baking mat.
- Toss butternut squash with oil, syrup, cinnamon, pepper, and salt. Spread evenly on the baking sheet and roast for 25 to 30 minutes, stirring occasionally.
- Place pecans on a piece of foil or small baking sheet and toast at 400F for 5 to 10 minutes or until fragrant, watching carefully.
- Assemble bowls. Divide rice between two bowls. Add greens, squash, apples, cranberries and toasted pecans.

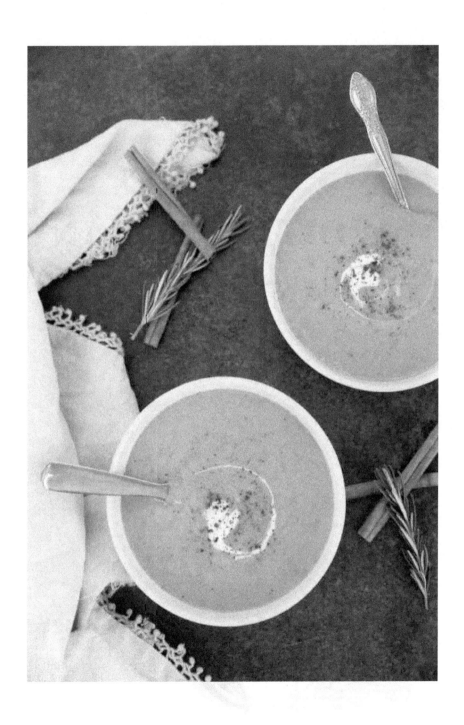

MEDITERRANEAN EGG AND RECIPIES

Mediterranean Feta & Quinoa Egg Muffins

INGREDIENTS

- 2 cups baby spinach, finely chopped
- 1/2 cup finely chopped onion*
- 1 cup chopped or sliced tomatoes {cherry or grape tomatoes work well}
- 1/2 cup chopped {pitted} kalamata olives
- 1 tablespoon chopped fresh oregano
- 2 teaspoons high oleic sunflower oil, plus optional extra for greasing muffin tins
- 8 eggs
- 1 cup cooked quinoa*
- 1 cup crumbled feta cheese
- 1/4 teaspoon salt

INSTRUCTIONS

- Pre-heat oven to 350 degrees fahrenheit, and prepare 12 silicone muffin holders on a baking sheet, or grease a 12 cup muffin tin with oil and set aside.
- Chop vegetables and heat a skillet to medium. Add vegetable oil and onions and saute for 2 minutes. Add tomatoes and saute for another minute, then add spinach and saute until wilted, about 1 minute. Turn off heat and stir in olives and oregano, and set aside.
- Place eggs in a blender or mixing bowl and blend/mix until well combined. Pour eggs in to a mixing bowl {if using a

blender} then add quinoa, feta cheese, veggie mixture, and salt, and stir until well combined.

- Pour mixture in to silicone cups or greased muffin tins, dividing equally, and bake in oven for 30 minutes, or until eggs have set and muffins are a light golden brown. Allow to cool for 5 minutes before serving, or may be chilled and eaten cold, or re-heated in a microwave the next day.

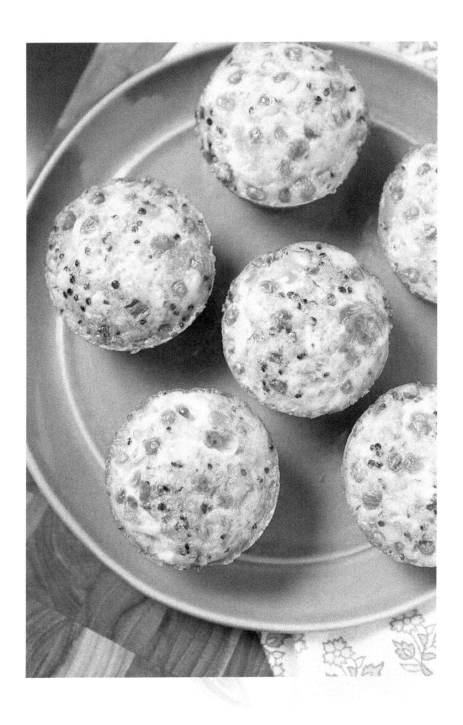

MEDITERRANEAN BREAKFAST BAKE

Swedish Breakfast Buns

Ingredients:

- 3/4 cup almond flour
- 1 Tbsp flax seeds
- 1 Tbsp sunflower seeds (shelled)
- 2 Tbsp psyllium husk powder
- 1 tsp baking powder
- 1/2 tsp salt
- 2 Tbsp olive oil (extra virgin, or light)
- 2 eggs
- 1/2 cup sour cream (or creme fraiche)

Instruction

1. Preheat oven to 400 degrees. Mix almond flour, seeds, psyllium, salt, and baking powder in a bowl. Add eggs, olive oil, and sour cream and mix it carefully. Let it sit for 5 minutes.
2. Cut the dough into 4 pieces. Shape into balls and put in a cake pan (I use a 9 inch circular pan, but anything really will work here so long as it has sides). Bake for approximately 20-25 minutes.
3. Enjoy!

Easy Almond Flax Keto Bread Recipe (Paleo & GF)

Ingredients

- 1 1/2 cups blanched almond flour
- 1/4 cup ground flax seeds
- 1 tbsp whole flax seeds
- 1/2 tsp sea salt
- 1/2 tsp baking soda
- 4 large eggs beaten
- 1/2 tsp apple cider vinegar
- 2 tsp honey (optional- omit for keto)
- 1 tbsp butter or oil, to grease the loaf pan

Instructions

1. Preheat the oven to 300°.
2. Mix all ingredients together (except for the butter--which is used to grease the pan) until thoroughly combined.
3. Grease an 8 or 9 inch loaf pan or just line it with parchment paper instead.
4. Pour dough into the loaf pan and bake at 300° for 45 minutes, or until a toothpick inserted into the bread's center comes out clean.
5. Cool before serving.

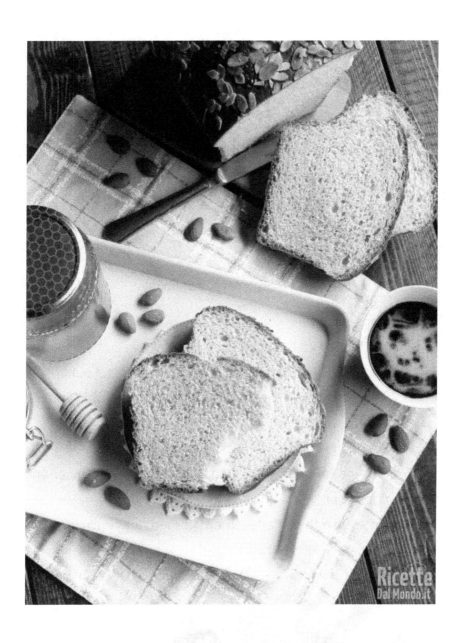

Coconut Flour & Psyllium Flatbread

Ingredient

- ½ cup Coconut flour
- 2 tablespoons Psyllium Husk powder
- 1.5 oz Coconut oil (or melted butter)
- ½ teaspoon Salt
- 1 teaspoon Baking powder
- 1 Cup Boiling water
- Herbs/garlic powder to flavour optional

Instructions

1. Mix the dry ingredients with a hand whisk.
2. Add the oil and blend well. It will look like a nut butter.
3. Add the boiling water, half at a time and blend until a dough like mixture forms.
4. Divide the mixture into 6 balls.
5. Roll the balls between 2 sheets of parchment paper and flatten out.
6. Either use them flattened or cut them into a circle with a saucepan lid.
7. Dry fry in a pan for 2– 3 minutes each side, until golden.

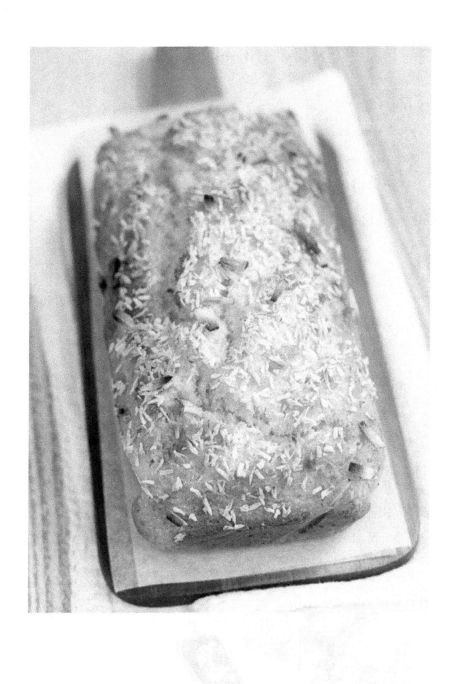

Holy Hotness Bread

Dry Ingredients

- 1½ cups flaxseed meal
- ½ teaspoon baking soda
- ½ teaspoon baking powder ¼ teaspoon sea salt

Wet ingredients

- ⅓ cup chopped tomato 1 serrano pepper
- ¼ cup chopped red bell pepper
- 11 cups fresh baby spinach (5–6 ounces) ¼ cup liquid egg whites
- 1½ teaspoons vinegar

Directions

1. Preheat the oven to 350°F.
2. Cover a 9 × 13-inch baking sheet with Pan Lining Paper, foil side down.
3. In a medium bowl, mix together the dry ingredients.
4. Blend wet ingredients thoroughly in blender.
5. Transfer the wet mixture to the bowl of dry ingredients. Mix well and quickly.
6. Scrape the batter onto the prepared baking sheet. Push the mixture to the edges, then level with a spatula. Bake for about 60 minutes or until dry to the touch.
7. Place upside down on a cooling rack. Remove the pan and paper. Let cool.
8. After cooling, cut into desired pieces or use as a prebaked pizza crust. Store in a sealed container in the refrigerator.

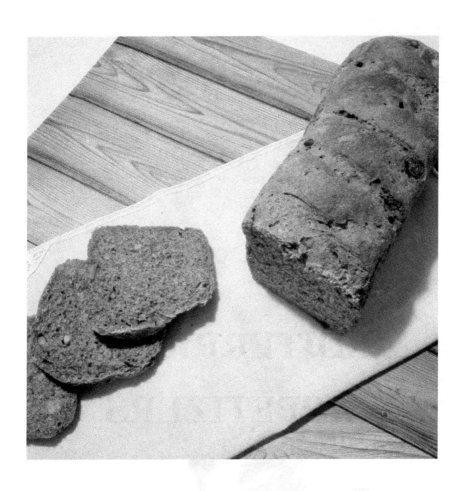

MEDITERRANEAN APPETIZERS

Tuna Spread

Total time: 15 minutes

Prep time: 15 minutes

Cook time: 0 minutes

Yield: 16 servings

Ingredients

- 1 shallot, chopped
- 1 (8 oz.) container cream cheese spread (chives-and-onion flavor)
- 1 tsp. Italian seasoning
- 1 hard-cooked egg, finely chopped
- 1 medium tomato, coarsely chopped
- 1 (6 oz.) can tuna, drained, cut into chunks
- ½ cup pitted Kalamata olives, halved
- 1 tbsp. chopped fresh parsley
- 48 crackers

Directions

- Mix together shallot, cream cheese, and Italian seasoning in a small bowl until well blended; spread the mixture on a serving plate.
- Top with egg, tomato, tuna, olives, and parsley and serve with crackers.

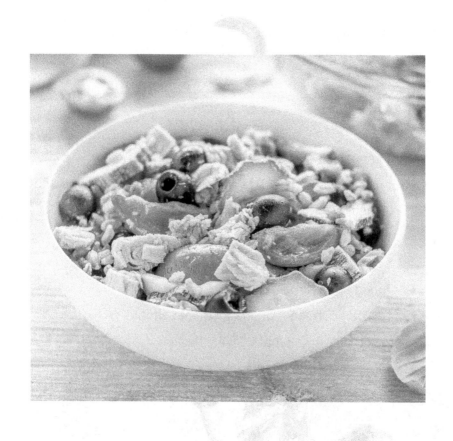

Mediterranean Salad Kabobs

Total time: 15 minutes

Prep time: 24 minutes

Cook time: 0 minutes

Yield: 24 servings

Ingredients

- ¾ cup nonfat plain Greek yogurt
- 1 small clove garlic, chopped
- 2 tsp. chopped oregano leaves
- 2 tsp. chopped dill weed
- 2 tsp. raw honey
- ¼ tsp. sea salt

Kabobs

- 12 slices English cucumber, halved crosswise
- 24 small grape tomatoes
- 24 pitted Kalamata olives
- 24 toothpicks

Directions

- Mix the dip ingredients in a small bowl and set aside.
- Thread half slice cucumber, 1 tomato, and 1 olive on each cocktail pick.
- Serve the kabobs with dip.

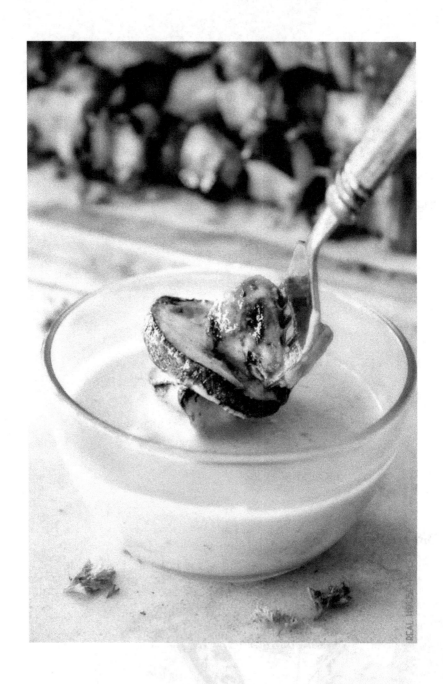

CPSIA information can be obtained
at www.ICGtesting.com
Printed in the USA
BVHW061948150621
609639BV00002B/588